Alternative Healing Boosters
PART 1 of 29: Aromatherapy

By **Larry J George**

I0493999

(Alternative Healer and researcher)
help@spiritopia.org
http://amazon.com/author/larryjgeorge

Learn to heal yourself with the various remedies from all around the globe.

No experience required!

Discover all remedies in the author's page on Amazon:
http://amazon.com/author/larryjgeorge

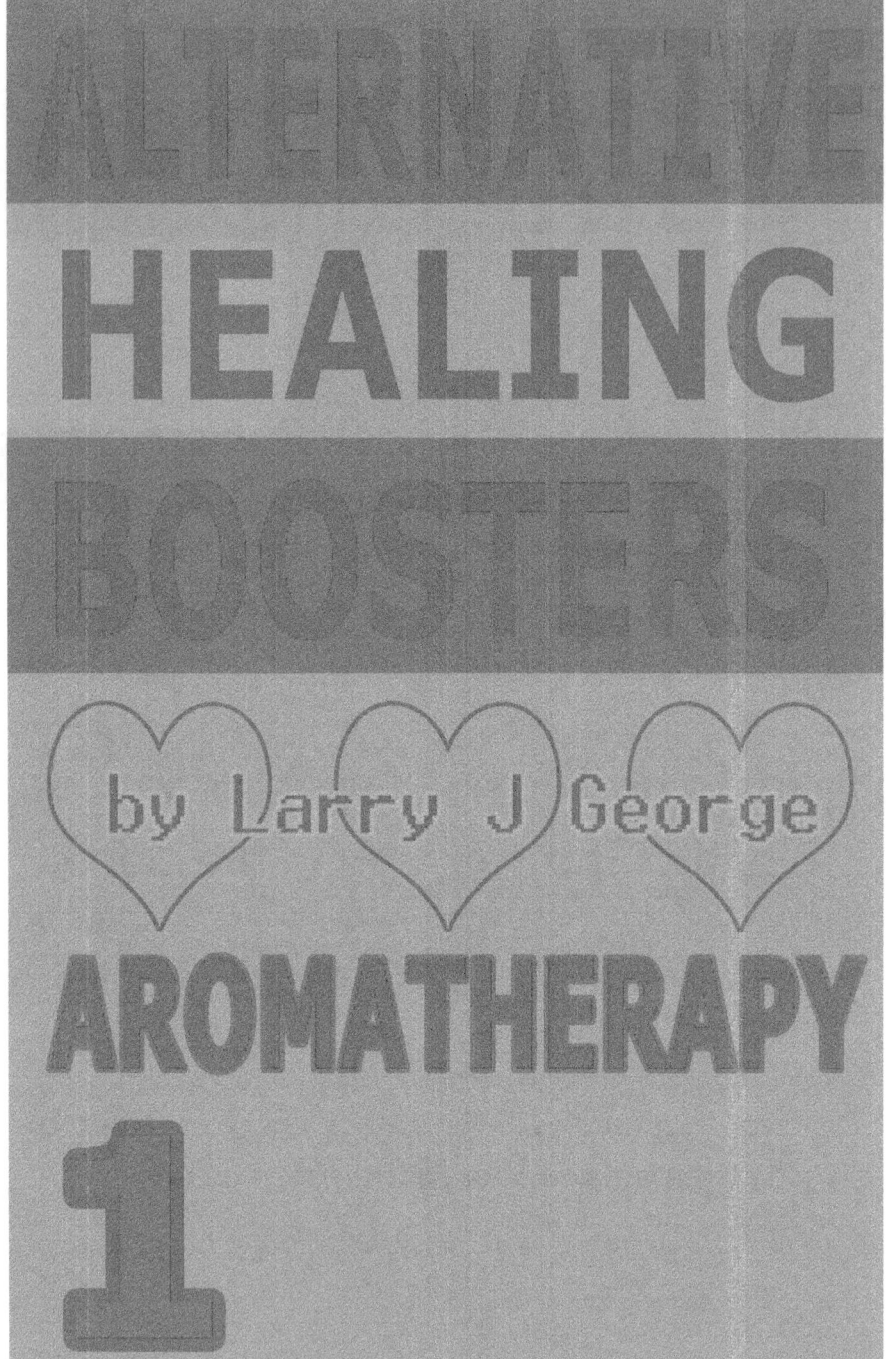

ALTERNATIVE
HEALING
BOOSTERS

by Larry J George

AROMATHERAPY
1

ISBN-13: 978-1499386301

ISBN-10: 1499386303

Disclaimer: Due to the nature of the book subject, the author cannot guarantee success with any of the alternative healing boosters (remedies). Although the author has put all his efforts to present accurate and valid information to the user, the tremendous growth of alternative healing remedies worldwide cannot allow us to offer any kind of success by applying what is mentioned in this book.

Printed by **CreateSpace**, An Amazon.com company

Table of Contents

Foreword

Aromatherapy is a word often associated with calm, sweet smelling and relaxing surroundings. It is famous for its mostly relaxing indulgent features and using aromatherapy has also been known to have medicinal qualities.

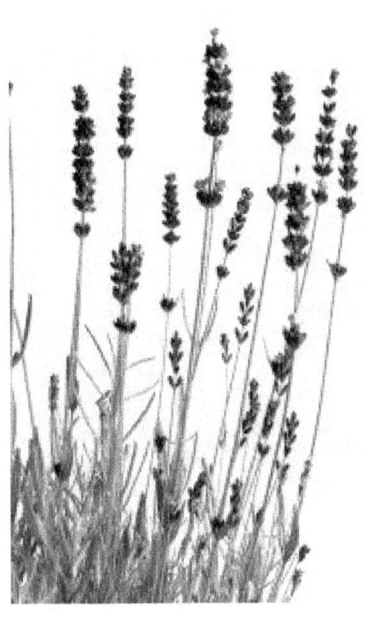

Aromatherapy Ambiance

Learn About The Healing Art Of Aromatherapy!

Chapter 1 - Aromatherapy- The Basics

The basis of aromatherapy lies in its use of naturally garnered essential oils. These oils are usually extracted from plant materials and other compounds. The flower based oils are usually used for strongly aromatic uses while the other sources of oils are mainly used for medicinal purposes. These oils are primarily extracted from flowers or delicate plant tissues which are well known for their various attributes.

Surprisingly, even in the culinary field, such elements are now becoming popular, especially among those with a more discerning palate. Also, it must be noted that such elements have long been used as a more traditional source of nutrition and even flavor.

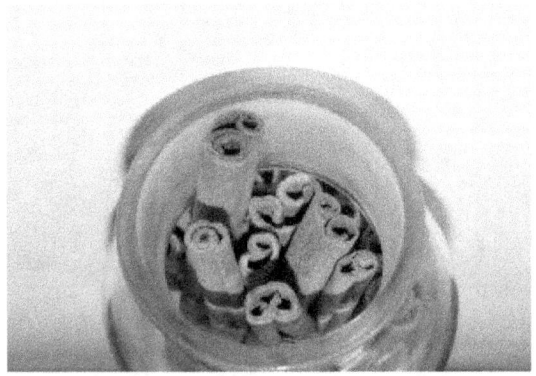

The Basics

Sometimes divided into three distinctive areas of uses, aromatherapy is proved to be an effective solution to many problems. Aerial diffusion falls in the category of environmental fragrancing or disinfection.

Direct inhalation is encouraged to arrest various respiratory problems like respiratory disinfection, congestion, tightness in the chest cavity, etc. Topical applications are mainly for relaxing purposes such as massages, baths, compresses and therapeutic skin care treatments.

Theoretically, aromatherapy is encouraged as an alternative to more invasive type of treatments. Besides being very pleasant as a treatment option, it can sometimes even be touted as a preventive element to certain diseases.

At worst, it can play a major role in relaxing the general state of an individual and perhaps can contribute in a better and more successful way to recovery when combined with other more scientifically accepted methods of treatment.

Today there are many avenues of treatment to explore before embarking on a particular type suitable for the individual. However it should also be noted that before making a choice, one must try to be as well informed as possible.

YOUR NOTES:

_____

_____

_____

_____

_____

_____

_____

_____

_____

_____

_____

Chapter 2 - Understanding Aromatherapy

The importance of understanding a particular topic, idea, or element is often overlooked in this busy world of today. It is often difficult to find the time to extensively explore the topics. However, with the use of various modern tools, this task can be not only fun but very informative too.

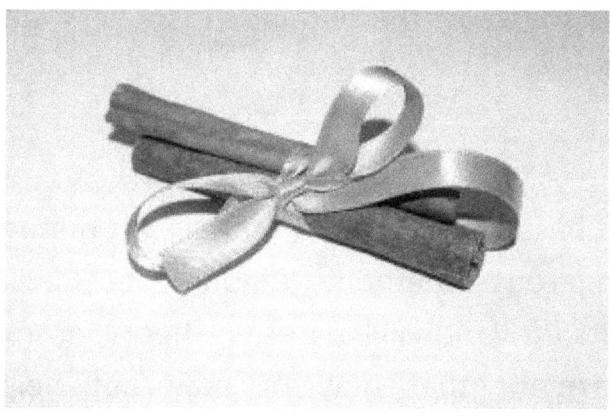

Digging A Little Deeper

Most people today regard aromatherapy as just another indulgent exercise which only privileged people enjoy.

However, after spending time to delve deeper, one is likely to find a whole new prospect related to the diverse uses of aromatherapy.

Aromatherapy can be explored as an alternative to more invasive methods of treatments. Originated long before medical science made discoveries and break-throughs; aromatherapy has had many success stories to back its wondrous attributes. The concept of using aromatherapy to treat wounds and burns first came about when a scientist badly burned his hand while conducting an experiment. Later, it was again used successfully as an antiseptic to treat the wounded soldiers during the world war two.

Since it is based on natural materials, aromatherapy is a less dangerous method, among the best suited treatments for various illnesses. In theory, aromatherapy is a treatment that may or may not help in the prevention of diseases by the use of essential oils. When coupled with the more conventional methods of treatments, it has been found to produce impressive results, mainly contributing as a calming ingredient to the equation.

Aromatherapy can have a positive impact on the limbic system through the olfactory system. It has also been known to have direct pharmacologic effects. Though many studies have been conducted to prove the connection of direct impacts of use of aromatherapy coupled with other scientific methods, but no conclusive data has been drafted to date.

YOUR NOTES:

_____

_____

_____

_____

_____

_____

_____

_____

_____

_____

_____

_____

_____

_____

Chapter 3 - Considering Aromatherapy

Some consider aromatherapy as a new age alternative style of treatment, while yet others know of its origins that date back a long while.

Indulging in aromatherapy is a choice that should only be made after understanding the various aspects of this field. This is most important when choosing aromatherapy as an alternative to medical treatments and when trying to arrest, cure or prevent diseases.

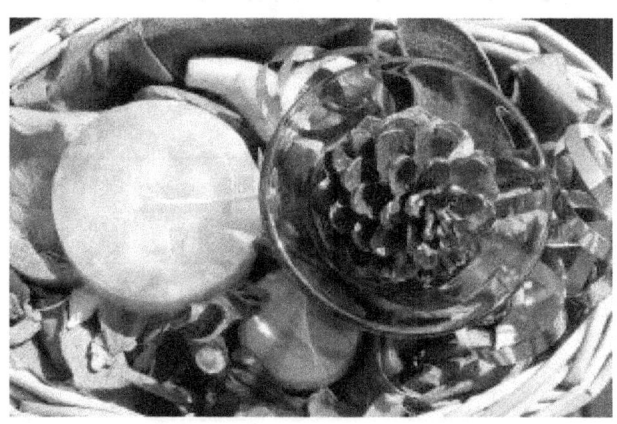

What To Think About

The general perception of aromatherapy is that the scent of essential oils is infused into the atmosphere to create a pleasing and relaxing state of body and mind. To others, it may be perceived as a relaxing massage session with the use of beneficial essential oils.

Using aromatherapy as a skin care regimen is also very popular. Many of the essential oils used have proven qualities that can contribute to the various needs for skin care.

These requirements can range from keeping the skin looking young and supple to actually reversing the aging effects on the skin. Some forms of eczema and acne have been successfully arrested with the use of the aromatherapy method. Aromatherapy is also an excellent way recommended to get oneself into a meditative state. These meditative states are usually associated with yoga, tai chi, visualization or self hypnosis.

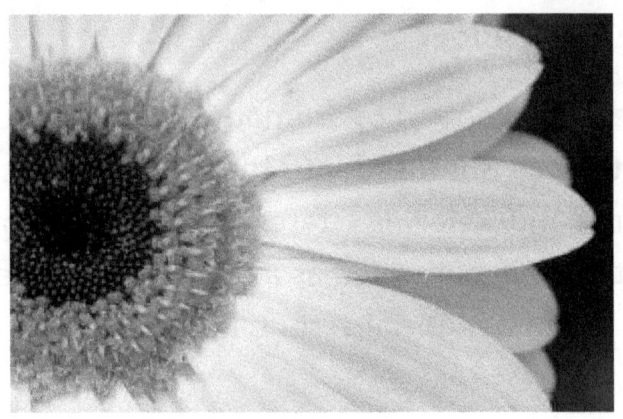

To reach the required level of meditation, sometimes various numbers of oils need to be tried.

Furthermore, some studies show that aromatherapy may help to create the mood for various scenarios with some definite results in mind.

It is a fact that large number of people switch to the use of aromatherapy even though there is no conclusive evidence that shows that aromatherapy is successful in treating certain diseases.

This is basically after listening to other people's success stories.

However, aromatherapy is a traditionally proven success in the treatment of emotional and physical ailments which is mainly because it helps the body in coping up with stress, anxiety and tension, all of which contribute or are the causes of other diseases and illnesses.

YOUR NOTES:

_____

_____

_____

_____

_____

_____

_____

_____

_____

_____

_____

_____

_____

_____

_____

_____

_____

Chapter 4 - Using Aromatherapy Effectively

Aromatherapy is fast gaining popularity. Though it is still primarily linked with providing relaxation and other therapeutic message sessions, other new uses of this field are also being explored.

Traditionally aromatherapy was used for almost everything starting from relaxing to health solutions and ending at culinary preparations. Before starting on this journey of using aromatherapy, a lot has to be understood and studied.

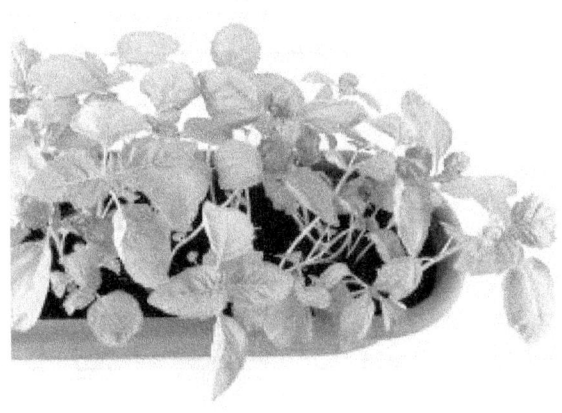

What You Need To Know

Before setting up of an aromatherapy centre or using aromatherapy to treat a specific medical condition, buying of the proper essential oils is an important aspect to be taken into consideration.

Because of commercialization most of the essential oils available in the market are not that genuine as they are stated on the labels. Careful examination is required and they need to be properly checked and rechecked before being purchased.

Some labels are also deceiving in the capabilities that they profess. The type of packing and its condition is also an important factor to be taken into consideration. There should not be any cracks or broken seals in the packing as this will lead to the contamination in the purity of the oils to be bought.

It is also to be noted that the best results are obtained only by the proper method and choice of the essential oils. This means that some essential oils work better and to the best of their abilities only when they are used the correct way.

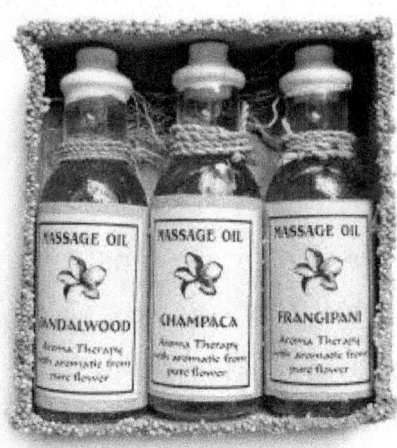

For the treatment of certain diseases like sinuses, headaches, colds, chest congestions, etc method of inhalation is used as it is more effective and quicker than other methods like oral or direct application on the skin.

While treating anxiety, depression, stress and other pressurizing conditions the method of spraying the essential oils and distilled water creates a calming and relaxing atmosphere.

While some conditions prefer spraying or inhalation, some conditions require direct application on the skin.

However, while doing this the concentration of the essential oils applied needs to be carefully monitored because these essential oils may induce allergic reaction in the patient.

YOUR NOTES:

_____
_____
_____
_____
_____
_____
_____
_____
_____
_____
_____
_____
_____
_____
_____
_____

Chapter 5 - More Ways Of Using Aromatherapy

Aromatherapy which is commonly believed to just consist of essential oils used for calming and therapeutic massage session is paving its way in other fields as well. These may include treating other medical conditions that have previous success rates from using aromatherapy methods.

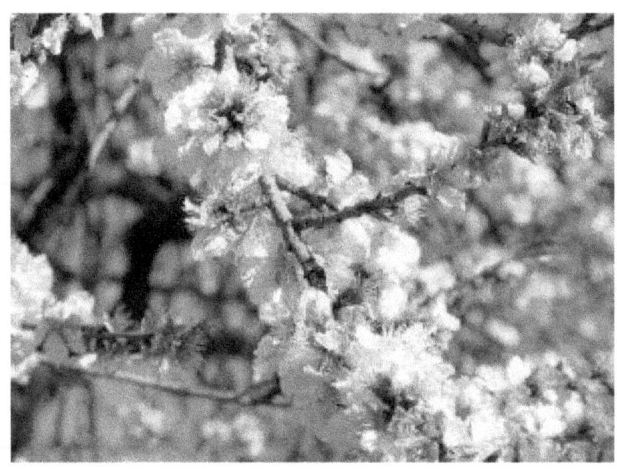

What You Can Do

Some cultures traditionally have used aromatherapy to treat wounds and scars successfully. For example, essential oils containing Helichrysum ingredient is used to repair damaged skin conditions.

Helichrysum has a strong anti-inflammatory and concentration of regenerative diketones and it is because of this fact that it is considered highly for treating damaged skin. It also has a pleasant earthy aroma which has a therapeutic effect.

Essential oils like lavender, rosemary and sage are also known for healing skin conditions. Small amounts of sage is effective in healing old scars and stretch marks but care should be taken regarding higher amounts as Thujone present in sage can be toxic.

Certain essential oils contain antiseptic elements and thus it is widely used t treat wounds. Tea tree essential oil is used to treat wounds and it is used until the wound is completely sealed and after that it is no longer needed.

Aromatherapy treatment may also be used for a healthy and younger skin. They get absorbed into the skin and provide all the necessary nutrients to the skin which makes it look healthy.

Besides skin care aromatherapy is used in bath salts, shower gels, shampoos and body lotions. These create the desired effects of sweet smelling and relaxing moods. Further aromatherapy in this form is mild and non-threatening in its purest form.

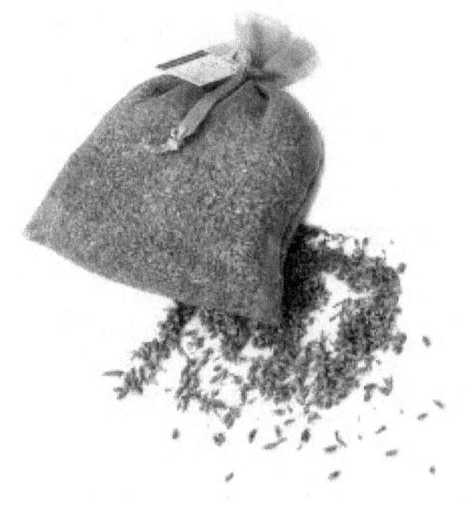

Essential oils like lavender have a calming effect on the mental turmoil state. They encourage the senses to slow down creating a peaceful mind which helps in relieving impatience and irritability.

Chapter 6 - Cures Using Aromatherapy

Approaching a medical condition by exploring the possibility of using aromatherapy as a solution is definitely worth the effort.

Aromatherapy ideally works by including and tackling the psychological and the physical aspects of a medical condition together. When these are taken into account all the contributing factors are studied first before any treatment is performed.

Before any recommendations regarding aromatherapy other factors like the medical history of the patient, his emotional condition, his general health and lifestyle are to be taken into consideration. This comes under holistic approach to treating a medical condition.

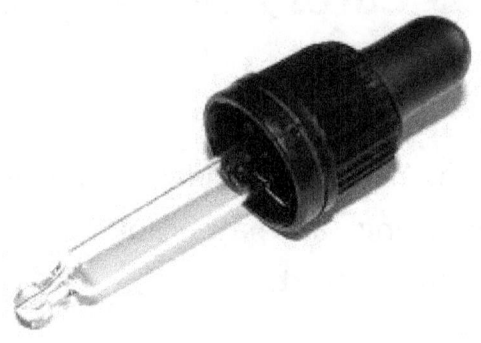

Applications

Other conditions that can be treated using aromatherapy include backaches, irritable bowel syndrome, headaches and depression, etc. A large percentage of the above ailments are due to stress. The aroma therapist after centering the patient's stress causing source can successfully treat the medical condition. in other extreme cases reports of complete recovery have also been documented.

Conditions like dermatitis, acne, eczema, psoriasis, cellulite, varicose veins, stretch marks and other skin conditions are known to be completely treated by the use of aromatherapy.

While other medical treatments may have undesirable side effects while combating depression, hysteria, lack of concentration and panic attacks aromatherapy is widely successful in these fields. Some essential oils have surprisingly quick and effective results while treating burns, bruises and sprains.

Asthma, bronchitis, flu, and muscular aches and pains are some other areas in which aromatherapy has been found to be successful. However, its success depends upon the proper choice of a qualified aromatherapy practitioner and the proper quality of the essential oils to be used.

YOUR NOTES:

_____

_____

_____

_____

_____

_____

_____

_____

Chapter 7 - Healing Attributes Of Aromatherapy

The widely popular beliefs that most illnesses and diseases are somehow linked to stress, anxiety and lack of proper daily nutrition have its own benefits.

It is advised to keep all the negative aspects of one's life under control even though it seems to be a bit unrealistic as some illnesses need to reach a critical stage before they are visible or can be detected.

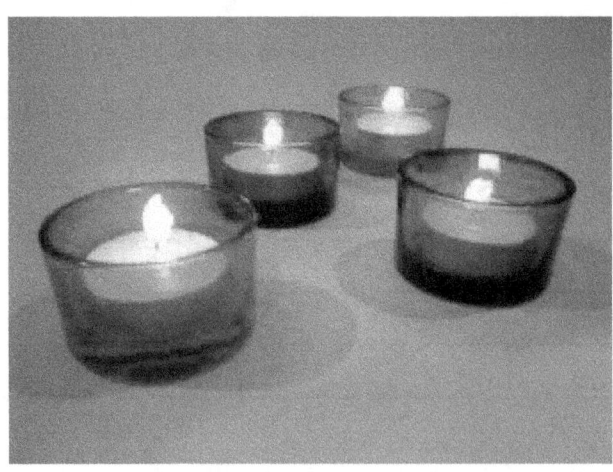

Wellness

Aromatherapy with its best use in producing a calming and soothing effect on the mind of a person can thus helpfully contribute to this end. Furthermore, there is also a huge list of other conditions that can be successfully treated using aromatherapy elements.

Below are just a few examples of the capabilities and merits of using aromatherapy:

* Acne – lavender oil or tea tree oil to be applied directly onto the affected area. For milder cases, using a body bath lotion with these properties is recommended.

* Anemia – a concoction of tincture from the yellow dock root or an extract of dandelion leaf or even eating dandelion greens as a salad.

* Anxiety – chamomile, California poppy, passion flower, lemon balm

* Asthma – ginkgo biloba, mullein oil, a Chinese herb called shuan huang lian

* Bee sting – urtica urens , cantharis, lavender and vegetable oil mixed

* Body odor – alfalfa contains chlorophyll.

* Cold – eucalyptus oil in boiling water and inhaled. Gargle with a mixture of tea tree oil

Cholesterol – chicory root, ginger

* Constipation – aloe vera juice, ginger tea

* Hair loss – saw palmetto, arnica, jojoba oil

* Headaches – chamomile relaxes, ginkgo biloba improves blood circulation

* Dandruff – flaxseed oil, primrose oil or salmon oil. Rinsing hair in chaparral or thyme

* Diabetes – huckleberry, tea made from most beans

* Diarrhea – blackberry tea, wild oregano

* Eczema – chickweed added to bath, stinging nettle, hazel ointment

* Indigestion – gentian root for better digestion, ginger, peppermint

* Nausea and vomiting – catnip leaves, chamomile flowers

* Menopause – for skin use geranium essential oil, orange blossom water, sandalwood essential oil

Chapter 8 - Aromatherapy And Healing

Aromatherapy is gaining huge popularity and has been taken seriously only recently as a feasible alternative treatment method to convectional medical remedies. However, it was practiced in most ancient cultures with successful results.

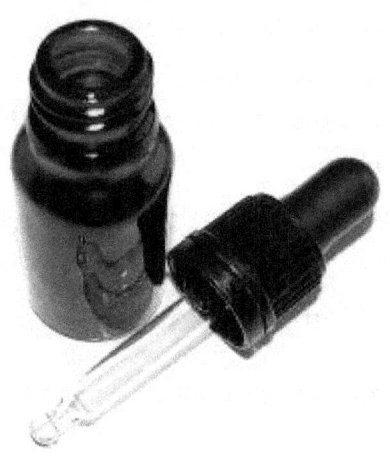

More In Depth Healing Info

Aromatherapy is widely confused in its attributes which is mainly due to the commercial sector who seeks to capitalize in this area. It is popularly believed to be linked to some pleasing scent that is emitted from some essential oils.

Aromatherapy is effective only on proper application and intent. It creates a positive impact on a person physically, mentally and spiritually which would further affect the body condition of the person.

What happens however in the commercial market is that the products are publicized to contain some essential oils for aromatherapy purposes but they do not contain them in the proper needed dosage and thus is not considered aromatherapy.

Aromatherapy is basically a practice of using essential oils for medicinal and therapeutic purposes. Some essential oils contain anti-viral, anti-fungal and anti-bacterial properties and thus are used remedial purposes. Some essential oils may help treat skin problems also.

Chapter 9 - Misusing Aromatherapy

Over the past years the term aromatherapy is been used in a completely wrong and misleading manner mainly due to commercial reasons that the mass population does not really know what does it mean.

It is basically a combination of two words- aroma and therapy, however many false claims have been made on it over the past years to promote and capitalize on it.

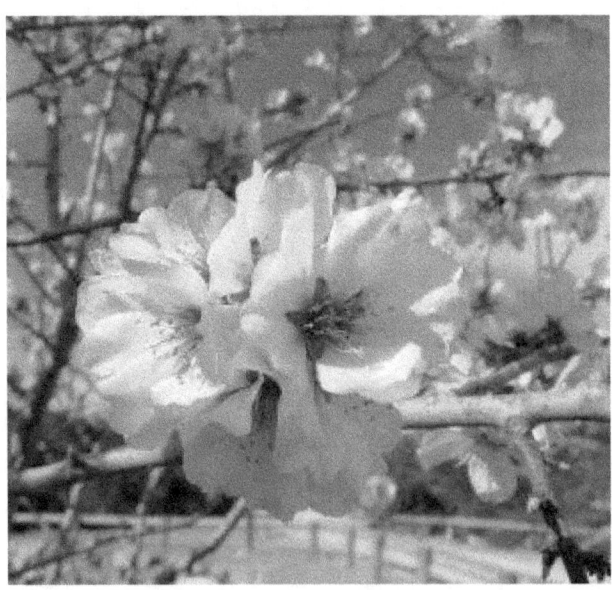

Be Cautious

Aromatherapy is a actually a very serious field as it involves the use of pure essential oils and other natural ingredients which are safe only if applied and used correctly, some essential oils also being toxic in nature. Without understanding and gaining knowledge of the oils and natural ingredients being used one should not pursue it as it may lead to some serious repercussions.

Pregnant women and lactating mothers should especially be very careful while using aromatherapy as the strong scent may be harmful to the babies as their senses and immune system is not fully developed yet. Some scents can also be off putting to the babies and may affect the baby's sleeping pattern and feeding schedule, causing health problems from the initial stages.

Even though it has a calming effect aromatherapy should always be used after seeking the doctor's permission because it may have some adverse effects on the patients. Some essential oils may have negative effects on the prescribed drugs that the patient may already be taking.

One should use aromatherapy as an alternative to other medicinal options only after conducting extensive studies on it and properly understanding all its advantages and disadvantages.

Treating a medical condition using aromatherapy may give minimal positive results to actually combating the disease even though stress and anxiety is found to be the root causes most of the diseases.

Overuse or overenthusiastic use of aromatherapy is seriously harmful especially when it is being used without proper medical advice. Some studies show little of no evidence in its effectiveness against bacterial, fungal or viral infections, thus proving it to be poor alternative against other medical practices.

Since in most countries aromatherapy is linked to just providing a relaxed and calm atmosphere, there is no regulatory body governing the use, content and potency of the essential oils in the aromatherapy session.

Improper use of essential oils and natural ingredients may cause some serious repercussions. Undiluted essential oils can cause skin irritation and discolorations while. When the natural products have been exposed to pesticides and other chemicals in their growing stage they may have many negative impacts on application. In presence of estrogen like elements there may be negative effect on the delicate skin of children.

Aromatherapy influence is taken by some cultures to the extreme. There is a widespread practice of ingesting certain ingredients which may cause severe irreparable damage. Medical advice should always be sought before use as some essential oils may also be toxic.

As with bioactive substances some essential oils even though they are safe for general public, they may still have adverse effects on pregnant or lactating women.

There may be adverse effects while using some ingredients and methods in a particular aromatherapy session when they are made to interact with other conventional medicinal elements. Adulterated oils can also pose a threat to health depending upon the type of substance used.

Finally unsubstantiated claims by those promoting aromatherapy as a proven alternative treatment may also be misleading and thus harmful.

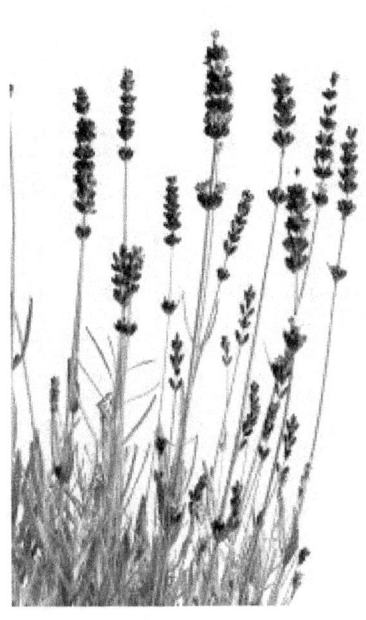

Chapter 10 - Acquiring Aromatherapy Products

Before undertaking aromatherapy for treatment purpose, one should take proper time and effort to understand the fundamentals of aromatherapy especially because aromatherapy and essential oils are linked up.

This effort is essential because it may lead to the wrong use of essential oils, their incorrect application or even the use of products that may not even contain any essential oils at all.

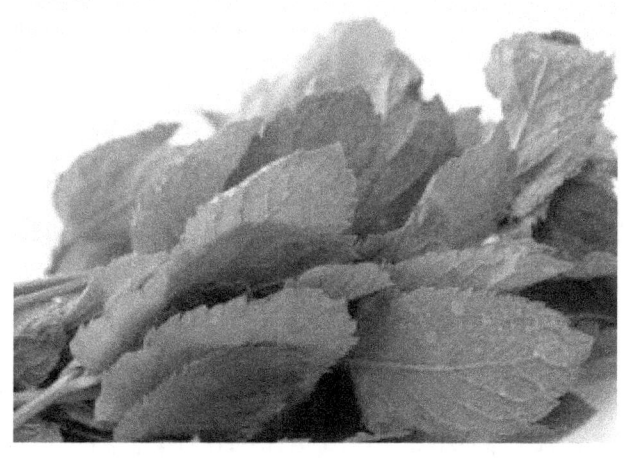

What's Good and What's Not

Proper care should be taken regarding the quality of oils used. Poor quality oils lack the optimum benefits that it promises to give.

Many factors need to be taken into consideration for example, if there are added chemicals or preservatives or some other substandard quality ingredients or whether they have been produced in poor processing environments or if there is any adulteration of oils.

Serious health damage may be caused if the above precautions are not taken into consideration and at best only minimal benefits can be derived from them.

Lesser grade ingredients may be added to the essential oils to attain higher profits. Words like fragrance oils, natural identical oil and perfume oil are misleading.

Without any strict guidelines some vendors use words like therapeutic grade or aromatherapy grade and thus these should be ignored and the products should be bought only after close examination.

Packaging styles are especially very misleading. Dark colored bottles may be a way by which the vendors may hide the purity of the oils inside.

Plastic packing is also not wise because of the reaction of plastic with some essential oils which may finally deteriorate the quality of the said oils.

YOUR NOTES:

_____

_____

_____

_____

_____

_____

_____

_____

Wrapping Up

Aromatherapy or the essential oil therapy is a natural and gentle way of treating disorders. It is also the least invasive medicinal treatment method. It may also be used as a compliment to some other treatment. Sometimes it may also serve as the only treatment regimen.

Aromatherapy is particularly beneficial to patients who are required to be in a non stressful state of body and mind mainly because of the calming and soothing atmosphere that it provides. Some studies show that inhaling some particular scents may immediately bring to rest the stressful nature of the patients which finally contributes to the given disease or illness.

We hope that this book has been beneficial to you and has given you an insight on how to make use of aromatherapy.

Bonus Blessings

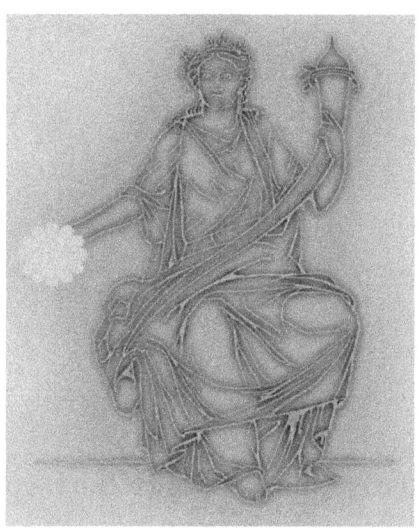

Receive some **free bonus blessings** by the Triple Goddess of Fortune. Just visit the link below, look at the image and receive the blessings (1 time/day).

Bring some positive energy into your life.

People have reported being energized after receiving the blessings. Others have reported a boost in self-confidence. Please don't over-use.

Thank you. Blessed be.-

RECEIVE FREE BLESSINGS CLICK:

http://spiritopia.org/fortune/

Bonus Astrological Profile

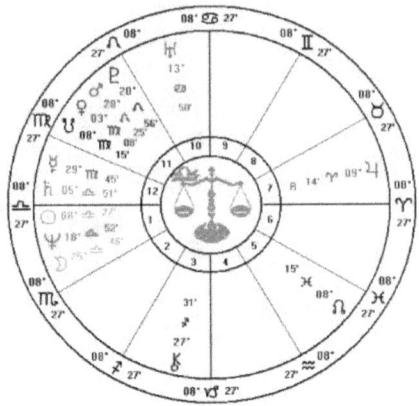

Would you like a totally free astrological profile derived from the ancient texts of Chinese astrology?

Get it here 100% free. Simply enter your birth details and wait for the profile to appear. Then you can easily print it or you can request a more advanced version for a small fee. Just go to this website:

http://astroprofile.us/

Bonus Spiritual Protection Shield

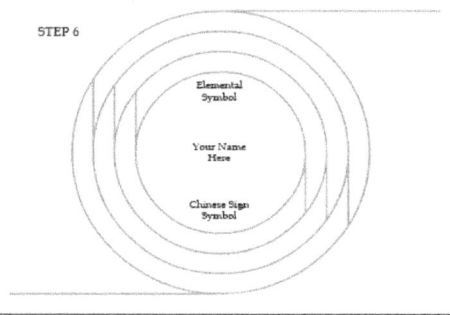

Are you suffering from negativity around you? Would you like to drive it away gradually and steadily? Then draw a Protection Shield in a piece of paper and start recycling negative energy to outer space. Visit the link below to see a representation of the shield in your browser (this is an animated gif image):

http://spiritopia.org/protection_shield.gif

If you want to learn how to draw this shield in an A4 size piece of paper using mathematical instruments like a ruler or a protractor, please visit the page below:

http://www2.chineseastrologer.org/protection_shield.php

Online Resources

So you want to explore more? Here are some resources that you might find helpful online:

http://en.wikipedia.org/wiki/Aromatherapy

http://spiritopia.org/supreme/1/

http://www.happymassage.com/wiki/Aromatherapy_Massage

http://spiritopia.org/supreme/2/

http://how-to.wikia.com/wiki/How_to_use_Aromatherapy

http://spiritopia.org/supreme/3/

END OF PART 1.

All the healing wisdom of the world in one place.-

GET ALL 29 PARTS FROM:

http://amazon.com/author/larryjgeorge

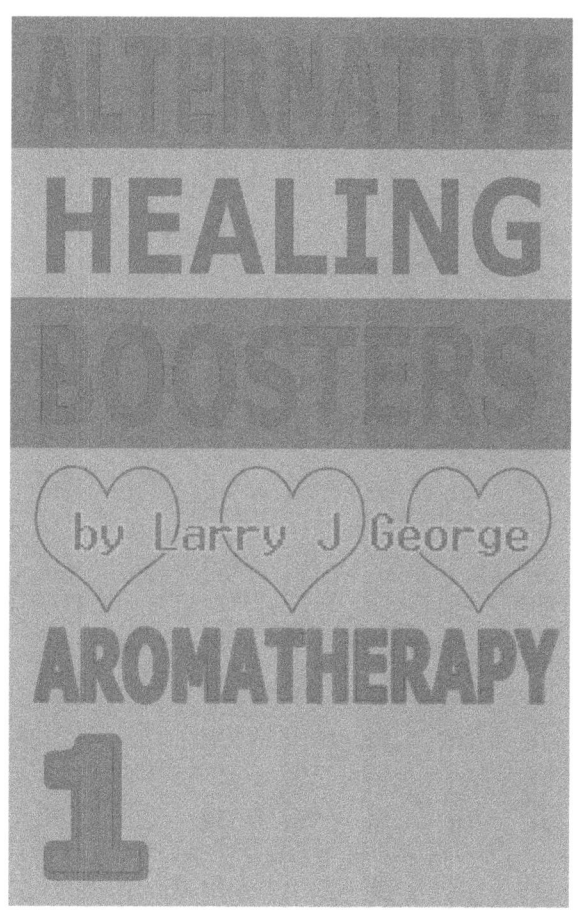

www.ingramcontent.com/pod-product-compliance
Lightning Source LLC
Chambersburg PA
CBHW070714180526
45167CB00004B/1474

* 9 7 8 1 4 9 9 3 8 6 3 0 1 *